Table of Contents

INTRODUCTION

On some level, most people know that eating nutritious meals ultimately equates to healthier living. It can start to get a little nebulous, however, when you're talking about optimal nutrition and what that means in the context of your overall health.

OPTIMAL NUTRITION VERSUS ADEQUATE NUTRITION

Every cell, tissue, and organ in the human body relies on nutrients for energy to perform its function properly. Nutrients come from the food you eat. In the best-case scenario, you eat a well balanced diet with lean meats, poultry, and fish along with lots of vegetables, legumes, fruits, and healthy nuts. This healthy diet provides nutrients such as minerals and vitamins, which become energy sources on a cellular level. In contrast, if you eat meals and snacks loaded with processed foods, salt, sugars, and fats, your body doesn't get what it needs to properly grow and thrive, which can compromise not only normal function, but also long-term health. Adequate nutrition refers to eating foods that provide the bare minimum for survival. For instance, it's possible to eat mostly junk food like salty potato chips, meals like high fat frozen dinners, and sugary snacks. In contrast, optimal nutrition means you're consistently eating foods that properly fuel your body for top performance.

7 Benefits of Optimal Nutrition

Optimal nutrition works on a variety of levels, providing mind, body, and spirit wellness benefits. These benefits also feed into each other, having a more profound impact on long-term overall health, enabling you to live a long, productive life.

1. Helps maintain a healthy weight

The most obvious health benefit of optimal nutrition is that it's much easier to reach and maintain a healthy weight. Avoiding being overweight or obese puts you on a healthy trajectory and lowers your risk of developing serious or life-threatening diseases and conditions.

2. Lowers risk for chronic conditions

Pairing optimal nutrition with making healthy lifestyle choices — exercising regularly and not smoking or excessively drinking alcohol — is a winning combination. It plays an important role in lowering your risk of developing chronic disease such as diabetes, heart disease, high blood pressure, and high cholesterol

3. Boosts natural immunity

Not only does optimal nutrition fend off chronic health conditions, but it also boosts your immune system. Eating plenty of fruits and vegetables — which are sources of nutrients such as selenium, iron, zinc, protein, and vitamins C and D — support the function and growth of immune cells

4. Improves healing and recovery from injury or illness

Many of the same nutrients that act as immunity boosters also come into play for wound healing. But that's not all. When your body is properly fueled with nutrients, it's better equipped to heal and recover more quickly from things like surgical procedures, illness, and injury.

5. Helps the digestive system function properly

Optimal nutrition also impacts your digestive system. Eating a balanced nutrient diet not only enhances healthy digestion, but it also staves away issues like irritable bowel syndrome. In fact, optimal nutrition is one of the best ways to enhance your digestion naturally.

6. Supports healthy muscles and strong bones

Getting optimal nutrition contributes to strong bones and healthy muscles, literally from your head to your toes. Strong bones rely on a steady stream of calcium and vitamin D found in dairy foods, green leafy vegetables, and fish. Food rich in protein and low in saturated fat builds healthy muscle.

7. Increases mood and energy levels

Remarkably, optimal nutrition also affects your mental health. When you properly fuel your body, your energy level rises and you simply feel better. So instead of reaching for that bag of chips or those fat laden cookies the next time you have a particularly challenging day, grab an apple, carrot, or a handful of natural almonds. Your body will thank you now and for years to come.

Do These Things Now to Keep Your Metabolism Strong Later

You're out enjoying a meal at a restaurant. While you're grazing through the fifth salad of the week, your rail-thin spouse is enjoying a big cheeseburger with a pile of greasy French fries. It just doesn't seem fair. If only there was a way to supercharge your metabolism today so you'd have a fighting chance of having a healthy weight as you age. Actually, that isn't as far-fetched as you may think. In this blog, the team at Cardio Metabolic Institute explains what you can do today for a stronger metabolism tomorrow.

Metabolism explained

You're no doubt familiar with the word. After all, at some time or another many people either blame a slow metabolism for weight challenges or become jealous over a friend's fast metabolism. But do you really know what metabolism is? As its name implies, metabolism refers to chemical or metabolic reactions that occur when your body takes the food and beverages you consume and converts it into the energy needed to operate – everything from breathing to making and repairing cells to establishing body temperature and virtually everything in between.

If metabolism sounds like a complicated and important process, it is. It not only occurs during every waking moment, but it's also operating when you're sleeping. Your basal metabolic rate (BMR) is a mathematical calculation that determines the baseline number of calories your body needs to perform the most basic, or basal, functions, such as breathing.

Numerous effects on metabolism

The rub with metabolism is that whether you have a fast or slow one is largely determined by gender and genetics as well as age. Research has shown that at about age 60, BMR begins to decline. Also, men generally have a higher metabolic rate than women because they typically have less body fat and more muscle, enabling them to burn more calories. The good news is that while you can't control genetics and age, there are plenty of things you can do today to boost your metabolism and keep it strong in the future. Spoiler alert! It's all about energy (food) and activity.

Eat healthy and drink more water

Do yourself a favor, and kick those processed foods, fried foods, and refined sugars to the curb. These types of foods are likely to end up being stored as fat. To boost metabolism, choose a healthy diet with plenty of lean protein, whole grains, and fruits and vegetables — foods your body can leverage to fuel its activities and functions..What's even better is that research shows that increasing protein in your diet has both short-term and long-term benefits. Diets higher in protein temporarily increase metabolism by about 15%-30%. In the long run, a protein-rich diet builds muscle mass. And people with more lean muscle mass tend to have a faster metabolism, which burns more calories. While you're eating healthier, don't forget to drink plenty of water throughout the day, which also helps your body burn more calories.

Get up and get active

When it comes to building new habits today to build a strong metabolism tomorrow, exercising and becoming more active are important. Similar to incorporating more protein into your diet, increasing physical activity has both short- and long-term advantages to boosting metabolism. Weight-bearing exercise — using resistance bands or lifting weights — builds muscle mass, which can burn calories even when your body is at rest. Aerobic exercise, like cycling, swimming, or even walking, is an efficient way to burn more calories.

Get adequate sleep

You probably know that getting a good night's sleep helps your body recover and restore and also lowers your risk for health complications like high blood pressure, diabetes, and having a stroke or heart attack. But did you know it affects metabolism? Problems sleeping may change the way your body uses glucose and can interfere with the hormones that regulate metabolism.

I'm At Risk for Heart Problems — What Should I Do?

On a typical day, you may come across multiple references to the term "heart healthy" — from the time you pour your cereal in the morning to notes on the restaurant menu at night and almost every moment in between. And for good reason. Heart disease is a leading cause of death in the United States, a dubious distinction it has held since 1950. In fact, each year about one out of every five deaths are due to heart disease. While the statistics are sobering, the good news is that a whopping 90% of heart disease can be chalked up to risk factors within your control, says the cardiovascular team at Cardio Metabolic Institute. In this blog, we take a look at lifestyle and modifiable factors to help you get more heart healthy.

Heart disease vs. cardiovascular disease
A great place to start unpacking this discussion is to clarify some terminology. Specifically, are heart disease and

cardiovascular disease the same thing?.While it may seem like these medical terms are used interchangeably, they're different. Heart disease is a catch-all name for the full spectrum of maladies that result in function or operational heart problems like heart attacks or congestive heart failure as well as physical issues with parts of the heart or vascular problems. Cardiovascular disease is a type of heart disease — in fact, it's the most common form. Cardiovascular disease includes the collection of conditions that result in blood flow problems to the heart that can result in heart attacks, heart failure, stroke, and peripheral artery disease.

Keep your blood pressure under control

When it comes to your heart health, blood pressure ranks as one of the most important risk factors you can control. High blood pressure is the No. 1 cause of heart disease and stroke because it damages the lining of your arteries, making them more vulnerable to the buildup of plaque, which ultimately narrows the arteries that lead to your heart and brain. Unlike other medical conditions, high blood pressure itself rarely has outward symptoms. So while half of all American adults have hypertension, many don't know it and only learn about their diagnosis after they suffer a heart attack or are being treated for an associated condition like kidney disease or a lingering leg ulcer that won't heal. Know your numbers. Get your blood pressure checked regularly, and seek treatment if it's not within normal range.

Eat a healthy diet

Not surprisingly, your nutrition plays a big role in your heart health. Good nutrition not only can mitigate your risk for heart problems, but it also does wonders for getting to and maintaining a healthy blood pressure. Think well-balanced meals with plenty of fruits, vegetables, and lean proteins. Just say no to fat-laden and processed foods as well as fried and salty foods. Our highly skilled registered dieticians at Cardio Metabolic Institute can help you create healthy meal plans and shopping lists and even provide healthy cooking tips.

Get up and get moving

What's particularly great about tackling the risk factors for heart issues is that the process tends to have a layered effect. So while you're doing things like eating healthier, getting active helps not only your heart health, but also your blood pressure.

Aim for about 30-60 minutes of exercise each day. Taking short walks, doing low-impact exercise like swimming, or even doing household chores like yard work counts. Find an activity that you enjoy, and stick with it. Not only does regular exercise help keep your blood pressure in check, but it also helps you maintain a healthy weight, which is a very good thing for your heart health.

Get a good night's sleep

While you may be more familiar with the importance of sleep in terms of your brain health and allowing your body and brain to refresh and restore, a good night's sleep also has an impact on your heart health. In fact, issues like sleep apnea have not only been connected to a higher risk of cardiovascular diseases, but also to all those risk factors that can result in heart issues like high blood pressure and poor diet choices.

If you're at risk for heart problems and want to learn more about steps you can take to mitigate your risk, contact Cardio Metabolic Institute. You can call the location near you — in Somerset, Monroe Township, East Brunswick or Edison, New Jersey — or book your appointment online today.

NUTRITION AND HEALTH: THE KEY TO WELL-BEING AND LONGEVITY

We all know that what we eat impacts our health and well-being. But many of us need to be made aware of how far that impact goes - not just in terms of the food we put into our bodies, but also the nutrients and energy it gives us. What if, for example, there was a way to unlock optimal performance simply by making certain dietary adjustments? Nutrition is critical to the preservation of welfare and good health. It is imperative for people to consume a diverse, balanced diet that comprises multiple nutritional components such as carbohydrates, proteins, fats, vitamins, minerals, and water. Fueling the body with this range of nutrients is essential for leading an optimal lifestyle. Here are some of the roles of nutrition in supporting good health:

Maximize productivity with Notion

Make a direct impact on our work while maximizing your productivity using Notion. Sign up now to unify your wiki, docs, and projects in one adaptive workspace. Start for free.

Heart Health

Eating a nutritious and balanced diet is essential for life, but it is also necessary for maintaining heart health. Our hearts work hard daily, pumping vital oxygen and nutrients throughout our bodies. To keep them performing optimally, we must provide them with quality nourishment following recommended dietary guidelines. Eating foods and drinks rich in antioxidants, fiber, and omega-3 fatty acids is critical to protecting our hearts. An anti-inflammatory diet centered around vegetables, fruits, legumes, and whole grains contributes to a healthier heart. This type of healthy eating aids in lowering cholesterol levels and reducing risk factors such as high blood pressure, ultimately leading to better overall cardiovascular health. So, we can ensure a healthier future by nourishing our bodies with good nutrition.

Bone and Teeth Strength

Nourishment is an essential part of having strong bones and teeth. Every meal, every sip you savor, every morsel you munch – every one of these actions impacts your bone and teeth health. That's why it's essential to understand nutrition's role in maintaining good bone and teeth strength. Thhe nutrients found in food provide our bodies with the building blocks required to create a strong skeletal structure that can withstand life's everyday demands. Eating the right foods will help replenish lost minerals and vitamins needed to maintain dental hygiene. Protein-rich diets are especially beneficial as they promote tissue growth and repair.

Calcium, crucial for healthy bones and cartilage, should also be included in a balanced diet. Additionally, foods containing Vitamin D, phosphorus, and fluoride further strengthen the construction of teeth by forming a protective layer..It's clear then that proper nutrition is vital to maintaining healthy bones and teeth. Eating suitable foods can prevent debilitating diseases such as osteoporosis and tooth decay and ultimately contribute to a longer and healthier life.

High Energy Levels

Eating healthy can be challenging, but it doesn't have to be. With the right vitamins and supplements, our bodies can function even better! We can increase our energy levels by taking in the proper nutrients and ensuring we get enough daily. Making smart food choices, such as foods rich in complex carbohydrates gives us sustained energy throughout the day while providing essential vitamins and minerals. Eating protein-rich foods helps build muscle and creates energy when combined with exercise..Choosing organic fruits and fruit juices, vegetables, and other natural products can offer additional health benefits, including antioxidants that prevent disease and illness. So let's start being proactive about nutrition and reap the rewards of increased energy and overall well-being.

Brain Health

There is increasing evidence that nutrition plays a crucial role in brain and mental health and function. A healthy diet can help support brain development and function and may even help to reduce the risk of certain brain disorders such as stroke, dementia, and Alzheimer's disease. A diet that includes fresh fruits, vegetables, whole grains, and lean proteins can provide the nutrients the brain needs to function correctly. These nutrients include vitamins, minerals, and antioxidants, which help to protect the brain from damage and support brain cell communication. In particular, research suggests that certain nutrients may be vital for brain health. For example, omega-3 fatty acids in fatty fish, nuts, and seeds may help improve memory and cognitive function. Similarly, B vitamins, which are found in whole grains, leafy greens, and animal products, may help to reduce the risk of brain disorders such as stroke and dementia.nLimiting your intake of unhealthy foods, such as those high in added sugars and unhealthy fats, is also essential, as these can negatively impact brain health. Additionally, it is essential to stay hydrated, as even mild dehydration can affect cognitive function. A healthy, balanced diet is important for maintaining good brain health and function.

Weight Control

Maintaining a healthy weight is imperative for overall wellness, and nutrition is essential in this process. The energy balance between the calories you consume and burn through metabolism and physical activity can be affected by what you eat and drink, meaning it's essential to select the right amounts of food for your age, gender, size, height, and exercise habits. Not only do calorie intake and portion sizes influence weight, but food and beverage choices also play a role. To stay full and satisfied, focus on nutrient-dense options like produce, whole grains, and lean proteins. Meanwhile, sugary drinks, unhealthy fats, and calories can lead to weight gain. Regular physical activity contributes to weight loss as well. A balanced diet filled with various nutrient-rich foods plus regular exercise is the key to achieving and keeping a healthy weight. Make sure to incorporate both into your lifestyle to live your best life. It all starts with minor changes.

Boosting Immunity

Good nutrition is essential for maintaining a healthy immune system.), as the nutrients in the foods and beverages we consume play a crucial role in the functioning of the immune system. A healthy, balanced diet that includes a variety of nutrient-dense foods can help to support the immune system and reduce the risk of illness. Several nutrients are essential for immune system function. These include:

Vitamin C: found in citrus fruits, strawberries, kiwi fruit, bell peppers, spinach, and Brussels sprouts

Vitamin E: found in nuts, seeds, and vegetable oils

Zinc: found in seafood, red meat, poultry, and beans

Selenium: found in Brazil nuts, tuna, and beef. In addition to these specific nutrients, a diet rich in fruits, vegetables, and whole grains can provide a range of antioxidants and other nutrients that can help support immune system function.

It is also important to pay attention to hydration, as proper hydration is essential for the immune system to function correctly. Finally, it is vital to get enough sleep, as sleep plays a crucial role in immune system function. A healthy, balanced diet that includes a variety of nutrient-dense foods, proper hydration, and sufficient sleep can help support a healthy immune system.

Digestive System Function

Good nutrition is vital for the proper functioning of the digestive system. The digestive system breaks down the foods we eat into smaller molecules that can be absorbed and used by the body for energy and nutrients. Several nutrients are essential for digestive system function. These include:

Fiber: found in fruits, vegetables, whole grains, and legumes. Soluble fiber can help to soften stools and promote regular bowel movements, while insoluble fiber can help to add bulk to stools and prevent constipation.

Water: essential for maintaining the proper consistency of stools and promoting regular bowel movements.

Probiotics: found in fermented foods such as yogurt, kefir, and sauerkraut. These beneficial bacteria can help maintain the gut microbiome's balance and support digestive health.

In addition to these specific nutrients, a diet rich in various fruits, vegetables, and whole grains can provide a range of other nutrients that can support digestive system function.

It is also essential to pay attention to portion sizes and to eat slowly, as this can help to promote proper digestion and absorption of nutrients. Additionally, regular physical activity can help support healthy digestion by stimulating food movement through the digestive tract.

Muscle Growth

Proper nutrition is essential for supporting muscle growth. For example, you create tiny tears in your muscle fibers when you exercise. To repair and grow stronger, your muscles need the proper nutrients. Protein is essential for muscle growth. It is the building block of muscle tissue and helps repair and regenerate damaged muscle fibers. You can get protein from various sources, including meat, poultry, fish, eggs, dairy products, beans, and soy. In addition to protein, your muscles need other nutrients to support muscle growth, such as carbohydrates and fats. Carbohydrates provide energy for your workouts, while fats help with hormone production and cell function.

It's crucial to consume enough calories to support muscle growth, but you should also be mindful of the types of calories you're consuming. A diet high in processed foods, added sugars, and unhealthy fats can undermine muscle-building efforts. To support muscle growth, it's a good idea to eat a balanced diet that includes a variety of whole, unprocessed foods. You should also pay attention to your protein, carbohydrate, and fat intake and ensure you're getting enough of each to support your workouts and muscle recovery.

Supporting Healthy Pregnancy and Breastfeeding

Nourishing your body correctly guarantees a sound pregnancy and breastfeeding journey. When expecting, females need extra sustenance to support the growth and development of their babies. Crucial nutrients to meet include Folic Acid, Iron, and Calcium. Folic acid reduces the risks of neural tube birth malformations, and Iron helps blood cells convey oxygen all through the body; calcium aids the advancement of bones and teeth. Moreover, during breastfeeding, moms require more calories to produce milk and similar nutritional values that sustain them throughout pregnancy. To ensure that mother and baby are healthy, strive for a balanced diet overflowing with whole foods. Last but not least, drink plenty of water and contact a healthcare provider or dietician if you need more clarification on nutrition.

Delaying the Onset of Aging

Proper nutrition may play a role in delaying the onset of aging. A healthy diet rich in various nutrients can help support overall health and well-being as we age. Some specific nutrients that may be important for aging include:

Antioxidants: These substances help protect cells from damage caused by free radicals and unstable molecules that can damage cells and contribute to aging and the development of chronic diseases. Good sources of antioxidants include fruits, vegetables, nuts, and whole grains.

Omega-3 fatty acids: These healthy fats have anti-inflammatory properties and may play a role in preventing the risk of heart disease, diabetes, and arthritis. Good sources of omega-3s include fatty fish, flaxseeds, and walnuts.

Vitamin D: This nutrient is essential for bone health and may also have other health benefits. Vitamin D can be synthesized by the body when the skin is exposed to sunlight, and it is also found in certain foods such as fatty fish, egg yolks, and fortified foods.

In addition to getting enough of these nutrients from various foods, it is also essential to eat a balanced diet low in added sugars, saturated and trans fats, and sodium. Maintaining a healthy weight and regular physical activity can also support healthy aging.

What to Know About Black Pepper and Piperine Supplements

Black pepper is a common spice used in cooking to enhance flavor. Pepper comes from the peppercorn, a dried unripe fruit. Peppercorns are picked when almost ripe and then allowed to dry until they turn black. Pepper contains piperine, an alkaloid that functions as an antioxidant. One teaspoon of black pepper provides 6 calories and 1 gram (g) of fiber.1 Piperine is also available in supplement form. Safety considerations: Safe when added to foods; as a supplement, piperine should be used with caution in people with diabetes, bleeding disorders, and gastrointestinal disorders. Piperine may interact with some medications.

Uses of Black Pepper

Supplement use should be individualized and vetted by a healthcare professional, such as a registered dietitian, pharmacist, or healthcare provider. No supplement is intended to treat, cure, or prevent disease. Black pepper is marketed for its anti-inflammatory properties. It is suggested to help with cognitive brain function and gastrointestinal function. It also has antimicrobial and antidepressant properties.

Yet, very few human clinical trials have assessed the outcomes of black pepper as a supplement. Below are some possible health benefits of black pepper. It should be noted that the studies reviewed mostly use a curcumin supplement combined with piperine. Curcumin is the active compound found in the spice turmeric. Therefore, it is not certain whether the results are due to one or both compounds. Additionally, most of the study outcomes focus on laboratory findings and not clinically significant findings like reduced risk of heart attack or secondary complications associated with diabetes. Therefore, the research is preliminary and not enough to recommend black pepper or piperine supplementation routinely.

May Lower Cholesterol Levels

Studies have looked at whether combining curcumin with piperine may have a role in improving lipid profiles which could prevent heart disease. A meta-analysis concluded that curcumin and piperine combined significantly reduced total and low-density lipoprotein (LDL) cholesterol (considered "bad" cholesterol) in people with metabolic syndrome. Another randomized, double-blinded, placebo-controlled trial evaluated the effects of 500 mg of curcumin capsules with piperine supplement in people with a previous heart attack.

After eight weeks, the supplement significantly reduced hemoglobin A1C, LDL cholesterol, and liver enzymes. It also significantly improved levels of high-density lipoprotein (HDL) cholesterol (considered "good" cholesterol). Although the results seem promising, the study populations were small, requiring future larger-scale trials to confirm the findings.

May lmprove Glucose Control

Combining curcumin and piperine may help lower glucose (blood sugar) levels in people with diabetes. Blood glucose control is important with diabetes to avoid further complications. Hemoglobin A1c (HbA1c or A1c) levels are measured over a three-month period in people with diabetes to assess the average glucose levels over the previous three months. In a small study of 71 participants, people were randomized to take either a placebo (an ineffective substance) or a supplement containing 5 mg of piperine and 500 mg of curcumin. After 120 days, those who took the supplement had significantly lower glucose levels, hemoglobin A1C levels, and levels of triglycerides (a fat in the blood). In people with type 2 diabetes, a daily dose of 500 mg of curcumin and 5 mg of piperine (compared to placebo) significantly reduced blood glucose, C-peptide, and A1c levels. The supplement also significantly lowered liver enzymes but did not affect C-reactive protein levels.

May Improve Liver Health

Metabolic dysfunction-associated steatotic liver disease (MASLD), previously known as nonalcoholic fatty liver disease (NAFLD), is a group of conditions with a fatty buildup in the liver. Common causes include obesity, insulin resistance, and diabetes.

A few studies suggest that piperine combined with curcumin as a supplement can improve liver function in people diagnosed with MASLD In one study, short-term treatment with curcumin and piperine seemed to reduce the severity of MASLD. Another study randomized 70 people with MASLD to receive a supplement of 500 mg curcuminoids with 5 mg piperine daily or a placebo for 12 weeks. At the end of the study, those who received the supplement had significantly lower concentrations of liver enzyme blood levels and less severe MASLD. Another study with a similar regimen in participants diagnosed with hepatic steatosis found that the supplement improved liver function enzymes and lipid profiles. However, it did not improve fibroscan measurements, which are used to assess the improvement of MASLD. Not many side effects are reported with the use of black pepper. Higher doses of black pepper may cause a burning sensation in the throat or stomach. It could also contribute to reflux or heartburn.

Precautions

Black pepper in amounts usually found in food is safe. Although safe in normal amounts, high doses of black pepper have not been studied for safety in pregnant people, breastfeeding people, or children. Lab studies have suggested that piperine, the chemical found in pepper, may slow blood-clotting.10 High doses could lead to bleeding. For this reason, you should discontinue piperine supplements for two weeks before any scheduled surgeries.

People with diabetes should monitor their glucose levels closely, as piperine can lower blood glucose levels. Adding piperine could reduce how much medication is needed. People with diabetes should discuss adding supplements to their regimen with their primary care provider to determine if medication dosage adjustments are needed.

People with gastrointestinal (GI) conditions, such as inflammatory bowel disease (IBD), may not tolerate pepper, but this can vary by person.

Dosage: How Much Black Pepper Should I Take?

There is no standard recommended dose for black pepper. Studies have shown that doses of piperine often range from 5 mg to 20 mg per day.3811 Five mg is usually the most common dose used in research studies. Always speak with a healthcare provider before taking a supplement to ensure that the supplement and dosage are appropriate for your individual needs.

Interactions
It's possible for piperine to interact with medications Some studies have shown that piperine can reduce blood glucose levels. Combining medications to lower glucose levels with piperine could theoretically lead to hypoglycemia. People with diabetes should always discuss supplements with their primary care provider or other treating provider before starting them. You may need to monitor your blood glucose levels closely.

Piperine may also slow blood clotting. Combining piperine with anticoagulant medications, such as Jantoven (warfarin), could increase your chances of bruising or bleeding as they have similar effects. Piperine can slow the breakdown of other medications in the liver, increasing the drug's effects. This may include:

Nonsteroidal inflammatory drugs (NSAIDs), such as Advil or Motring (ibuprofen)

Lipid-lowering drugs, such as Zocor (simvastatin)

Fexofenadine, such as Allegra or Mucinex Allergy

However, studies on these interactions were done in animals and used higher-than-normal piperine doses. Piperine could increase how the body absorbs some medications, including:

Phenytoin

Propranolol

Rifampin

Theophylline

Amoxicillin

Carbamazepine

Theoretically, this could increase the effects and possible side effects of these medications. It is essential to carefully read the ingredients list and nutrition facts panel of a supplement to know which ingredients and how much of each ingredient is included. Please review the supplement label with your healthcare provider to discuss any potential interactions with foods, other supplements, and medications.

How to Choose the Best Nut Butter for You

While adding any nut butter to your diet can offer health benefits, some nut butters are better suited for people with certain health conditions or dietary needs. Nut butters are a staple in many households, offering a satisfying, convenient, and nutrient-packed addition to toast, desserts, and bowls of oatmeal. But the number of nut butter options today can be overwhelming. Do you go for a classic peanut butter? Is almond butter healthier? If you are new to the nut butter scene and want to know which choice you should stock in your own pantry, keep reading to learn all about the wide variety of these protein-packed spreads.

The Best Nut Butter Choice for Every Situation

Nut butters are pastes made by grinding nuts. In some cases, other ingredients, like sugar, salt, cinnamon, and even chocolate are added to the mix. What was once a world dominated by peanut butter is now sprinkled with a wide variety of spreads, including hazelnut, pistachio, cashew, walnut, and pecan. Basically, any nut can be ground into a paste. "Nut butters make a great addition to a balanced diet because they provide heart-healthy fats, protein, and fiber," Liz Shaw, RDN, CPT, told Verywell. All nut butters will provide plant-based protein, healthy fats, antioxidants, vitamins, and minerals—some more than others.

The "best" nut butter depends on various factors, including taste preferences, dietary needs, financial situation, and health goals. And while each nut butter will fit into a balanced and healthy diet, some choices are "better" than others for certain individuals. As a rule of thumb, just remember to opt for nut butters that are free from excessive amounts of added sugar, salt, and other ingredients that may not support your health goals.

Pistachio Butter: Best for an Antioxidant Boost

Pistachio butter is made from the naturally colorful pistachio, and it provides a mild flavor and boost of nutrients. Pistachio butter is rich in healthy fats, including monounsaturated and polyunsaturated fats, as well as essential vitamins and minerals like potassium, magnesium, zinc, and copper. One factor that makes pistachios unique is their high antioxidant capacity. In fact, the antioxidant capacity of pistachios rivals that of popular antioxidant-containing foods,1 including blueberries, pomegranates, cherries, and red wine. Free radicals can cause harm to healthy cells, and over time, this damage may contribute to inflammation. This effect may speed up aging at the cellular level while potentially promoting heart disease and certain cancers.3 Consuming antioxidant-rich foods like pistachio butter (and pistachios!) may help protect cells from free radical damage in the body.

Walnut Butter: Best for Heart Health

Walnuts are the only tree nut that are an excellent source of alpha-linolenic acid (ALA), the plant-based omega-3 essential fatty acid.4 And between being a source of this healthy fat along with fiber, plant-based protein, antioxidants, and key micronutrients, walnuts (and hence walnut butter) are a heart-healthy food, especially when it is enjoyed as a part of an overall healthy and balanced diet.

Specifically, walnut consumption has been linked to a reduction of LDL "bad" cholesterol when enjoyed every day for two years, according to a study published in Circulation.

According to the American Heart Association, walnuts are especially high in omega-3 fatty acids, which are heart-healthy fats. A serving size is a small handful or 1.5 ounces of whole nuts or 2 tablespoons of nut butter.

Cashew Butter: Best for Iron Deficiency

Approximately 10 million people are iron deficient in the United States, including 5 million with iron deficiency anemia.7 People with iron deficiency can experience symptoms that include fatigue, headache, and even hair loss. While sources of heme iron will likely be your best bet to combat iron deficiency, like lean beef, including plant-based sources of iron in your diet may offer some benefits as well. Among the nuts out there, cashew butter tends to be one of the top sources of iron per serving. Just keep in mind that, like all nuts, cashews contain compounds that may negatively affect iron absorption, so you should not solely lean on this nut butter for all your iron needs.

Peanut Butter: Best for an Economical Nutritional Boost

Peanuts are the main ingredient in the most popular nut butter, and the perfect pairing for a sweet and fruity jelly spread. When it comes to bang for your buck, peanuts may be your best bet for nut butter selection.

One jar of peanut butter can sell for as little as $3 and change, which is far less than many other varieties, like almond and cashew.

Cost aside, peanut butter is a nutrient-packed spread that contains healthy fats, protein, vitamins, minerals, and unique plant compounds.

Almond Butter: Best for Blood Sugar Balance

Almond butter packs more fiber compared to many other but butter varieties, Shaw said. In fact, when compared with classic peanut butter, almond butter provides significantly more of this satiating nutrient, with more than 3 grams of fiber per each 2-tablespoon serving vs. 1.6 grams of fiber provided by an equivalent serving of peanut butter.

Fiber can help manage blood sugar since consuming it doesn't lead to a blood sugar spike. And data shows that a high-fiber diet can often improve blood glucose control. Almond butter also provides healthy fat and plant-based proteins, two other macros that help support healthy blood sugars.

Dietitians say that people can stay hydrated not only by drinking water but also by eating fruits and vegetables that are high in water content. Strawberries, watermelon, cantaloupe, lettuce, celery, and spinach are great examples of fruits and vegetables that can help you meet your hydration needs. While fruits and vegetables can support hydration, experts say that eating fruits and veggies alone is not enough to stay adequately hydrated. While drinking water is probably the most common way to quench your thirst, eating fruits and vegetables and drinking other types of liquids like smoothies and broths can also help you stay hydrated. "Hydration needs can be met through a variety of sources in addition to drinking water," Candace Pumper, MS, RD, LD, a registered dietitian at The Ohio State University Wexner Medical Center, told Verywell. "Raw fruits and vegetables also contribute to fluid needs because of their high water content." But there's a limit to how much fluid fruits and vegetables actually give you. Here's which ones nutrition experts recommend you add to your day to meet your hydration needs.

Why Hydration Matters

Staying hydrated helps your body with important jobs like regulating body temperature, protecting your joints, and getting rid of waste. Not drinking enough water can lead to dehydration, which can give you muscle cramps, dry mouth, tiredness, fatigue, headaches, rapid heart rate, and low blood pressure. If it's severe enough, dehydration can cause kidney damage, organ failure, brain damage, and even death.

How Much Water Do You Get From Eating Fruit?

According to Catalina Ruz, RDN, a registered dietitian at Top Nutrition Coaching, nutrient-dense fruits like strawberries, watermelon, and cantaloupe are refreshing and delicious sources of hydration. "Fruits can absolutely count as part of hydration due to their high water content. Several are incredibly hydrating as they contain over 90% of water," said Ruz. "Additionally, fruits are naturally sweet which can appeal to individuals who are less likely to consume enough plain water." Your daily water intake comes from both liquids and foods—including fruits and veggies with high water content. However, Pumper said that food generally only contributes about 20% of your body's total water intake. In other words, you only get about 20% of the water you need each day from the foods that you eat. Hydration doesn't need to be dull. Consider your preferences and add some hydrating fruits and veggies to your plate.

Even though fruits contribute water to your day, Pumper said that you would probably find it hard to stay hydrated just by eating fruit. "Fruits can assist in supporting hydration and may also be slightly, but not significantly, more hydrating than water in the short-term," said Pumper. "This is likely due to the electrolytes typically found in fruits that further benefit body fluid balance. However, Pumper also noted that your body's daily hydration status is generally well maintained as long as there is fluid and food available and balanced in your diet. "While fruits often get a bad reputation due to their sugar content, they are wonderfully rich in vitamins and can make hydration more enjoyable. For example, fruit is a rich source of vitamin C, folate, and potassium—vitamins that support the immune system, help maintain healthy vision, and act as anti-inflammatory agents against disease.

Can Vegetables Hydrate You?

According to Ruz, fruit isn't the only food with a high water content: adding vegetables to your diet can also boost hydration. Some veggies are over 80% water—think lettuce, cucumbers, cabbage, celery, spinach, and cooked broccoli. It is important for us to meet some of our hydration needs through fruits and vegetables but also consume water throughout the day. "Individuals consuming a diet rich in fruits and vegetables may not need to drink as much water due to these foods' water content Along with helping you meet your daily hydration needs, Ruz said that veggies are also a source of potassium as well as essential vitamins, minerals, antioxidants, and fiber. Plus, they're also naturally low in salt (sodium). "A potassium-rich diet can aid in cellular hydration and prevent water retention associated with a sodium-rich diet," said Ruz. "Therefore, a diet that consistently includes a variety of fruits and vegetables can absolutely help meet hydration goals."

Which Fruits and Veggies Are Most Hydrating?

Pumper said there are many fruits and veggies that are high in water content—it's all about finding which ones you enjoy the most.

Hydration Content of Fruits and Vegetables

Produce   % Water Content

Cucumbers   96

Celery 95

Radishes   95

Tomatoes   95

Zucchini and summer squash 95

Lettuce94–96

Asparagus   93

Bell peppers   92–94

Cauliflower   92

Mushrooms (white)   92

Kiwi   84

Source: USDA

How to Add More Fruits and Veggies to Your Diet

Ruz and Pumper also offered a few tips on how you can fit more of those super-hydrating fruits and veggies into your diet:

Add fruits or vegetables to your water. Drop a few slices of strawberries and cucumbers into your water bottle to make your drink more flavorful.

Eat veggies with your favorite dip. Pair hydrating snacks like carrots and celery with a tasty dipping sauce or spread (like ranch or hummus).

Make a smoothie. Use spinach, strawberries, bananas, and ice to make a nourishing and hydrating drink to give you energy throughout the day and help you stay hydrated.

Sprinkle fruits or veggies in your meal. You can add fruit to oatmeal or dry cereal for breakfast and top salads or soups with vegetables for lunch and dinner.

Is Eating Fruits and Veggies Enough to Stay Hydrated?

While some fruits and vegetables can help quench your thirst, Ruz said that they should not be a replacement for water or be the only things that you consume to stay hydrated. "It is important for us to meet some of our hydration needs through fruits and vegetables but also consume water throughout the day. Pumper said there are beverages other than water you can drink that count toward hydration—for example, teas, coconut water, homemade agua fresca, broths, and smoothies. If you choose to drink juice, Pumper recommends sticking with 100% juice and portions of 4 fluid ounces to keep calories in check. "Balanced eating means we are not solely relying on one food group or item for adequate nourishment," said Ruz. That said, "hydration doesn't need to be dull. Consider your preferences and add some hydrating fruits and veggies to your plate."

Eating fruits and vegetables with a high water content like watermelon, strawberries, celery, and spinach can be a good way to help you stay hydrated this summer. However, experts say these foods should not be the only way you meet your hydration needs. Consider drinking water throughout the day or other hydrating beverages like teas, coconut water, broths, and smoothies.

How Should You Consume Maca Root for Its Health Benefits?

Maca root comes from a vegetable grown in Peru and is sold in the US as supplement. It is touted for its adaptogenic properties and is said to boost energy and libido. Research is limited but some experts say maca is safe for most people. However, pregnant people should avoid maca due to potential lead exposure. Maca root comes from a plant native to Peru and has a culinary history going back almost 2,000 years. Traditionally cooked and used in soups or juices,1 maca eventually made its way to the United States as a superfood supplement.

Health food stores sell raw maca root powder and gelatinized maca root capsules with claims that these products can support energy, memory, female fertility, and more.1 It's considered an adaptogen and is said to help the body deal with stress.n"Maca root is something I use most often when caring for women, and for health needs specific to women.

Some older research suggests that maca may improve mood2 or treat antidepressant-induced sexual dysfunction in women,3 but most studies on maca were conducted on animals. "Animal-based research indicates maca root supports balancing of estrogen and progesterone. This may be why some women see benefit to fertility, and some experience relief from menstrual, perimenopause, and menopause symptoms when they take maca root. But there's not enough research to confirm the benefits of maca root.4 For those who want to take maca root for fertility issues, Khamba said they should speak with a provider to discuss whether it's appropriate. "Because maca root is a food, the risks associated with consuming it are low," Khamba said. "However, it's important to know that when any food is derived into powder or capsule form, it can be more concentrated than it is in its most natural state."

Maca Root Powder vs. Capsule: Does It Matter?

Maca is mostly sold in the U.S. as a powder or capsule. Some may prefer the capsule form since raw maca can have a strong, bitter taste, but the benefits are likely the same. "It probably doesn't make much difference how you consume it. Often, when in capsule form, maca root is combined with something else. So, I have a slight preference for mixing it into your food. The U.S. Pharmacopeial Convention says that "as a dietary supplement the recommended dose range is 1.5–3 g."5 "Generally, starting with smaller doses is best. Maca root works best when its effects are cumulative and happen over time.

FEEL GOOD FOODS: THE DIET-BRAIN CONNECTION

The diet-brain connection is a subject also referred to as nutritional psychiatry, the gut-brain connection, or "food and mood." It means that what we eat directly impacts our brains, and ultimately, our moods. The brain functions best when it is given high quality foods that nourish it, such as those containing vitamins, minerals, and antioxidants. Certain foods act as an aid in the "prevention and treatment of mental disorders," like depression.[1]

Our diet's impact on mental health might also impact appetite control and gut health.[1] Researchers have discovered that gut hormones are involved in the diet-brain connection.[2] These hormones are sent from the gut to the brain and contribute to cognitive functioning. The diet-brain connection is also crucial for the prevention of chronic illnesses. Most Americans' diets consist of high amounts of sugar, carbohydrates, calories, and fats, leading to diabetes, Alzheimer's disease, heart disease, and obesity.1

Diet's contribution to cognition goes beyond memory and processing speed and significantly impacts brain development. "During the development of brain structures in prenatal and perinatal phases, it is important that all the necessary energy and nutrients can be absorbed from the diet. This means that diet's influence on the brain begins before birth, as the infant is nourished by the mother's nutrients, and this impact on brain development continues throughout childhood.

Feel-Good Foods

Foods beneficial to mood are considered "feel-good foods" or "brain foods."1 Below you will find foods of different food groups that promote excellent brain health.

Fruits & Vegetables

Fruits and vegetables are essential supplements for optimum health. They not only nourish the body but the brain as well. Their properties contribute to psychological well-being,3 cognitive processing, and emotional regulation.2 Some carry more psychological benefits than others, which can be challenging to remember. So, experts found it fit to establish a memorable way to ensure that children and adults consume a balanced intake of different fruits and vegetables.

"Eat the Rainbow" Method

A dietary term referred to as "eat the rainbow" or "eat by color" is based on the concept that fruits and vegetables offer nutritional benefits depending on their color.bFor instance, purple and blue fruits and vegetables significantly benefit cognition and mood. The National Health and Nutrition Examination Survey (NHANES) found that 8 out of 10 Americans do not meet their daily requirements for all colors of vegetables and fruits.3 Purple and blue colors are the most neglected; 88% of people do not meet the appropriate daily consumption. Blueberries are a particular fruit that receives recognition as brain food. They exhibit cognitive benefits, especially throughout aging, during the stages of child development and cognitive decline.4 Their benefits are present even in small amounts. There are many other fruits, and veggies experts identify as brain foods.

Examples of purple and blue fruits and veggies are below:

Fruits

Blueberries

Blackberries

Purple grapes

Purple passion fruit

Plums

Prunes

Black currants

Elderberries

Figs

Vegetables

Eggplant

Beets

Ube (purple yam)

Purple cabbage

Purple carrots

Purple potatoes

Purple radish

Nuts

Nuts carry nutrients that are beneficial for brain health. They also have anti-aging properties and help preserve cognition in older age.5 Researchers examined the influence of "long-term intake of nuts" on older women's cognition.

Seafood & Eggs

Seafood consumption supplies many essential nutrients to the brain.7 Most seafood contains PUFAs, primarily omega-3 fatty acids, "especially eicosapentaenoic (EPA) and docosahexaenoic (DHA)." Fish, for example, are known to be rich in omega-3 fatty acids. Of all foods, fish is one of the most saturated with both DHA and EPA. They also are a great source of protein, which is necessary for brain health .Researchers evaluated diet during pregnancy, noted "breastfeeding duration," and examined their neurodevelopment at the age of four. It was determined that a diet including moderately high fish consumption (2-3 times a week), not other seafood, enhanced neurodevelopment for breastfed children for at least six months.10 However, according to the authors, further investigation is needed regarding seafood intake and child development.

Both eggs11 and seafood7 provide prenatal and early child benefits because of the positive effects that PUFAs have on cognitive development.7 However, pregnant women need to limit their seafood intake and avoid raw seafood altogether. Although too much seafood can cause "neuro-toxin contamination," there are prevalent neurodevelopmental benefits from consuming a limited amount of seafood during pregnancy.10 This is why a doctor typically recommends that a woman take a prenatal vitamin with DHA during pregnancy, to help with neurodevelopment and cognitive development. Eggs, like seafood, have omega-3 fatty acids and other types of PUFAs. They are also full of vitamins like folate, vitamin D, iodine,7 vitamin E, B12, and vitamin A.9 In addition, eggs are high in protein and contain lipids—another type of fatty acid.

Diets That Benefit Brain Health

There are still debates on the nutritional necessity for food groups other than fruits, vegetables, and nuts, like dairy, grains, legumes, and meat.3 Researchers have, however, found that diets that involve a balanced consumption of these food groups do offer brain health benefits. Diets that consist of vegetables, fruits, nuts, and other food groups that benefit overall health are recommended for a healthy brain-gut connection.bSome of these diets are listed below:

Mediterranean diet: Incorporates monounsaturated fats (MUFAs), like olive oils. This diet also includes mostly vegetables, fruits, grains, nuts, fish, and plant proteins.1 The Mediterranean diet also consists of reducing the consumption of red meats and refined sugar and grains.

This type of diet offers benefits for gut health and disease prevention. The Mediterranean diet additionally reduces cognitive decline.

The ketogenic diet (Keto): The Keto diet has recently become a popular source for "short-term weight loss."[1] This is a low-carbohydrate diet, that includes high amounts of fat and moderate protein. Animal studies have provided evidence that this diet does offer cognitive benefits.

The DASH (Dietary Approach to Stop Hypertension) diet: This is a low-fat and low-sodium diet, that includes a lot of PUFAs and consists of lean meats, poultry, fish, whole-grain cereals, nuts, fruits, vegetables, and low-fat or non-fat dairy products.[1] A research study found long-term effects of the DASH diet to result in better cognition. Researchers suspect combining the DASH diet with The Mediterranean diet to have the most cognitive impact.

Benefits of Feel Good Foods
There are various benefits of consuming foods that are considered "feel-good foods" or brain foods, such as:

Help prevent neurological disorders and mental illness

Contribute to brain development

Enhance cognition (memory, processing speed, and focus)

Establish mental clarity

Reduce brain fog and mental fatigue

Reduce anxiety and depression

Regulate emotions

Contribute to hormonal balance

Enhance immunity

Offer anti-inflammatory properties

Lessens the risk of chronic diseases

Increase energy

The foods mentioned above are scientifically recommended for the general public. These foods may not suit you, possibly due to allergies, health concerns, or dietary restrictions. If you are concerned about implementing any food into your diet, speak with your physician before doing so. Also, remember that every diet isn't for everyone. Find what is best for you and offers the benefits that you are searching for. It is equally important that you try not to judge yourself during transitioning into different dietary habits. Developing a new lifestyle habit is a process that takes time to establish. These foods can offer many benefits for your mental, cognitive and physical health, but it is difficult to incorporate every brain and mood-boosting food into your daily diet. Therefore, it is essential to be practical when attempting to have a more well-balanced diet. Not every day will be fully packed with "feel-good foods," and you do not have to feel bad about that. Start slowly—try adding one feel-good food to one of your meals today. Maybe tomorrow, you try out a different feel-good food and see how that goes. Try to stay curious about what foods taste good, feel good, and work for you.

CONCLUSION

Proper nutrition is essential for supporting a variety of different health goals. A healthy diet rich in various nutrients can support muscle growth, pregnancy and breastfeeding, and healthy aging. Eating a balanced diet that includes a variety of whole, unprocessed foods and paying attention to your intake of key nutrients such as protein, carbohydrates, fats, and antioxidants are essential. It is also important to stay hydrated and to talk to a healthcare provider or a registered dietitian if you have any concerns about your nutrition.